METABOLIC RESET DIET

2024

Stop Storing Fat, Balance Hormones and Lose Weight Naturally by Eating More Food Through Delicious Recipes and Easy 7 days Meal Plan

Andrew H. Steve

About the Author

Andrew H. Steve, a renowned nutrition and health expert, specializes in empowering individuals over 40 to reclaim their health. With a passion for nutrition and a deep understanding of the human body and metabolism, Andrew has successfully guided many to achieve significant weight loss and enhanced well-being.

With over a decade of experience, Andrew's approach is far from one-size-fits-all. He tailors his advice to each individual, focusing on a holistic method that encompasses a balanced diet, mindful eating, and an active lifestyle, rather than just diets and restrictions.

Known for his ability to distill complex dietary concepts into practical, actionable strategies, Andrew is a guiding force in navigating the intricacies of metabolism and wellness. His dedication extends beyond his professional achievements, as he finds joy in outdoor activities, experimenting with new recipes, and engaging in healthy discussions.

If you're looking to lose weight, increase energy, or improve your overall well-being, Andrew H. Steve is your ideal mentor. Under his guidance, you're not just adopting a healthy lifestyle; you're embarking on a transformative journey to rediscover your vitality and thrive.

TABLE O F CONTENTS

CHAPTER 1

INTRODUCTION

Introduction to the Metabolic Reset Diet 2024: A Revolution in Health and Well-being

In the ever-evolving landscape of health and wellness, the Metabolic Reset Diet emerges as a beacon of hope and transformation in 2024. This revolutionary approach to nutrition and lifestyle has captured the imagination of health enthusiasts and experts alike, promising not just weight loss, but a comprehensive overhaul of metabolic processes for enhanced vitality and well-being.

Overview of the Metabolic Reset Diet: Unveiling the Blueprint for Metabolic Harmony

Picture this: a personalized roadmap to unlock the hidden potential of your metabolism, restoring it to its optimal state. The Metabolic Reset Diet is not just another fad; it's a carefully crafted strategy that understands and adapts to the unique intricacies of your body's metabolic functions. It's a journey towards metabolic harmony, where the body becomes a finely tuned orchestra, playing the symphony of health.

At its core, the Metabolic Reset Diet focuses on resetting and recalibrating the body's metabolic rate. It goes beyond conventional dieting norms, acknowledging that each individual's metabolism is as unique as a fingerprint. This diet is not a one-size-fits-all solution; instead, it's a dynamic and adaptive approach that tailors itself to your body's specific needs.

Purpose and Goals of the Diet in 2024: Redefining Wellness in the Modern Age

In the year 2024, the purpose and goals of the Metabolic Reset Diet extend far beyond the pursuit of a slimmer figure. It is a holistic commitment to well-being, encompassing physical health, mental clarity, and sustained energy levels. The primary objective is not merely to shed pounds but to foster a profound transformation from within, addressing the root causes of metabolic imbalances.

As we navigate the complexities of modern life, our bodies often bear the brunt of sedentary lifestyles, processed foods, and stress. The Metabolic Reset Diet in 2024 aims to reverse this trend, offering a reset button for our metabolic systems. It strives to re-establish a harmonious relationship between the body and the nutrients it receives, with an emphasis on nourishment rather than deprivation.

Beyond weight management, the goals include improved insulin sensitivity, enhanced energy utilization, and a reduction in inflammation. The Metabolic Reset Diet is designed to empower individuals to take charge of their health, providing the tools and knowledge needed to foster lasting well-being.

Historical Context and Evolution of the Metabolic Reset Diets: Tracing the Roots of a Wellness Revolution

To truly grasp the significance of the Metabolic Reset Diet in 2024, we must delve into its historical context and evolution. The concept of metabolic resetting is not a recent phenomenon; it has roots in ancient practices that recognized the interconnectedness of diet, lifestyle, and health.

Ancient healing traditions, from Ayurveda to Traditional Chinese Medicine, underscored the importance of balance in all aspects of life. These age-old philosophies acknowledged that imbalances in the body's systems, including metabolism, could lead to various ailments. Fast forward to the present day, and we witness a convergence of ancient wisdom and modern science in the Metabolic Reset Diet.

The evolution of this approach reflects a growing understanding of the intricate dance between genetics, environment, and lifestyle choices. Advances in nutritional science, coupled with a wealth of data from metabolic research, have paved the way for a more nuanced and individualized approach to resetting our metabolic clocks.

As we stand on the precipice of a new era in health and wellness, the Metabolic Reset Diet of 2024 represents the culmination of centuries of wisdom and cutting-edge scientific discoveries. It is not merely a trend; it is a paradigm shift in how we perceive and prioritize our health, inviting us to embark on a transformative journey towards a revitalized and balanced life.

CHAPTER 2

FOUNDATIONS OF THE METABOLIC RESET DIET

In the intricate web of human physiology, the Metabolic Reset Diet serves as a compass, guiding individuals toward a profound understanding of their body's metabolic intricacies. As we embark on this journey, it's crucial to lay down the foundations, delving into the basics of metabolism and unravelling the scientific underpinnings of the Metabolic Reset Diet.

Understanding Metabolism

Metabolism, often dubbed the body's engine, is a dynamic and multifaceted process that orchestrates the conversion of food into energy, enabling the various physiological functions essential for life. Understanding metabolism is akin to deciphering the intricate dance of molecular reactions that sustain us. In this section, we'll explore the basics of metabolic processes and the factors that wield influence over this intricate symphony.

Basics of Metabolic Processes

At its core, metabolism involves two primary processes: anabolism and catabolism. Anabolism is the constructive phase, where the body synthesizes complex molecules from simpler ones, requiring energy. This is the process responsible for building and repairing tissues, such as muscle. On the flip side, catabolism is the destructive phase, involving the breakdown of complex molecules into simpler ones, releasing energy. This phase is crucial for extracting energy from the food we consume.

Central to these processes is the role of enzymes, the catalysts that facilitate and regulate metabolic reactions. Enzymes act like skilled conductors, orchestrating the biochemical reactions necessary for the body's functions. The intricacy of this molecular ballet is astounding, involving countless pathways and checkpoints to ensure optimal functioning.

The body's primary source of energy is derived from macronutrients – carbohydrates, fats, and proteins. Carbohydrates are broken down into glucose, fats into fatty acids, and proteins into amino acids. These building blocks are then utilized to generate adenosine triphosphate (ATP), the energy currency of cells.

Mitochondria, often referred to as the powerhouse of cells, play a pivotal role in energy production. Here, the process of oxidative phosphorylation takes place, extracting energy from nutrients to form ATP. The efficiency of this energy production process is a key determinant of metabolic health.

Factors Influencing Metabolism

Metabolism is not a static entity; it's subject to a myriad of influences that can tip the scales toward efficiency or sluggishness. Genetics, age, gender, and body composition all play roles in determining an individual's metabolic rate. Let's break down these factors:

- ***Genetics:*** The genetic blueprint we inherit contributes significantly to our metabolic profile. Some individuals may inherently possess a faster or slower metabolism based on their genetic makeup.

- ***Age:*** Metabolic rate tends to decrease with age, primarily due to a decline in muscle mass. This makes weight management more challenging as we get older.

- ***Gender:*** Men and women may experience differences in metabolic rate. Men generally have a higher muscle mass, contributing to a higher metabolic rate compared to women.

- ***Body Composition:*** Muscle tissue is more metabolically active than fat tissue. Therefore, individuals with higher muscle mass tend to have a higher basal metabolic rate (BMR).

- ***Hormones:*** Hormones play a crucial role in metabolism regulation. Thyroid hormones, insulin, cortisol, and others intricately modulate various aspects of metabolic processes.

Understanding these factors sets the stage for appreciating the uniqueness of each individual's metabolic landscape. The Metabolic Reset Diet recognizes this individuality, tailoring its approach to address the specific needs and challenges of each person's metabolism.

The Concept of Metabolic Reset

The Metabolic Reset Diet is not a mere compilation of dietary guidelines; it's a paradigm shift in how we perceive and interact with our body's metabolic processes. This section unveils the scientific basis of the Metabolic Reset and explores its profound implications for weight loss and overall health.

Scientific Basis

At the heart of the Metabolic Reset lies the concept of metabolic flexibility – the body's ability to seamlessly switch between energy sources and efficiently utilize different macronutrients. In modern society, where our diets are often skewed towards excessive carbohydrates and processed foods, our metabolic flexibility can become compromised.

The diet leverages the science of nutrient timing and composition to restore metabolic flexibility. By strategically combining macronutrients and timing meals appropriately, the Metabolic Reset Diet aims to recalibrate the body's reliance on glucose and encourage the efficient utilization of fats for energy.

Intermittent fasting, a key component of the Metabolic Reset Diet, further contributes to this flexibility. By incorporating periods of fasting, the body is prompted to tap into stored fat reserves, fostering fat adaptation and improving metabolic resilience.

Research on intermittent fasting and metabolic health is robust, highlighting its potential benefits for insulin sensitivity, inflammation reduction, and even longevity. The Metabolic Reset Diet draws inspiration from this body of evidence, weaving it into a comprehensive strategy for metabolic rejuvenation.

Relationship with Weight Loss and Health

While weight loss is often a primary motivator for individuals exploring the Metabolic Reset Diet, its impact extends far beyond shedding pounds. This dietary approach acknowledges that sustainable weight management is intricately linked to overall health and metabolic well-being.

The Metabolic Reset Diet's emphasis on balanced nutrient intake, coupled with intermittent fasting, creates an environment conducive to fat loss without compromising muscle mass. Unlike traditional diets that may lead to muscle depletion, the Metabolic Reset prioritizes the preservation of lean body mass, contributing to a more toned and metabolically active physique.

Beyond aesthetics, the diet addresses key markers of metabolic health, such as insulin sensitivity and blood sugar regulation. By promoting a balanced and diverse nutrient intake, it seeks to reduce the risk of metabolic disorders such as type 2 diabetes and metabolic syndrome.

In essence, the Metabolic Reset Diet redefines the relationship between food, metabolism, and health. It's a departure from restrictive and unsustainable diets, offering a sustainable and science-backed approach to not only transform bodies but to optimize the intricate processes that govern our vitality.

CHAPTER 3

PRINCIPLES AND GUIDELINES

Welcome to the heart of the Metabolic Reset Diet – the chapter where we unpack the fundamental principles and guidelines that will serve as your compass on this transformative journey. This is not just a diet; it's a comprehensive approach to reset your metabolism, redefine your relationship with food, and ultimately, revitalize your entire well-being.

Core Principles of the Metabolic Reset Diet

In this section, we'll delve into the core principles that form the backbone of the Metabolic Reset Diet. These principles aren't just rules to follow; they are the guiding lights that will help you understand and harness the power of metabolic reset.

Nutrient Composition

At the heart of metabolic reset lies a profound understanding of the nutrients that fuel our bodies. It's not just about the quantity of food; it's about the quality and balance of the nutrients you consume.

Macro Matters:

- **Proteins:** Your body's building blocks. Aim for lean sources like poultry, fish, tofu, and legumes.

- **Fats:** Opt for healthy fats found in avocados, nuts, and olive oil. These fats play a crucial role in hormone production and satiety.

- **Carbohydrates:** Choose complex carbs – whole grains, fruits, and vegetables – for sustained energy and fiber.

Micro Magic:

- **Vitamins:** Ensure a rainbow of fruits and veggies to cover your vitamin spectrum.

- **Minerals:** From calcium for bone health to iron for energy, diverse foods mean diverse minerals.

Hydration Station:

- Water is your ally. Stay adequately hydrated; it's the simplest yet often overlooked key to metabolic balance.

Meal Timing and Frequency

Timing is everything, especially when it comes to resetting your metabolism. The Metabolic Reset Diet places a strong emphasis on when and how often you eat.

Balanced Timing:

- **Breakfast Boost:** Kickstart your metabolism with a balanced breakfast within an hour of waking.

- **Lunch Logic:** Aim for a satisfying lunch around midday to maintain energy levels.

- **Dinner Dance:** Opt for a lighter dinner, allowing your body to wind down for the night.

Snack Smartly:

- Strategic snacks can keep your metabolism humming between meals, but choose wisely.

Intermittent Fasting:

- Explore intermittent fasting as a tool for metabolic reset. Experiment with fasting windows that suit your lifestyle.

Dietary Guidelines for Metabolic Reset

Now that we've explored the core principles, let's dive into the nitty-gritty of what to eat, what to avoid, and how to control your portions to make the most out of the Metabolic Reset Diet.

Recommended Foods

The Green Light List:

- **Vegetables:** A rainbow of colours ensures a variety of nutrients.

- **Lean Proteins:** Chicken, fish, tofu, legumes – choose your protein adventure.

- **Healthy Fats:** Avocado, nuts, seeds, and olive oil are your friends.

- **Whole Grains:** Quinoa, brown rice, and oats provide sustained energy.

Fruits in Moderation:

- While rich in vitamins, be mindful of the natural sugars in fruits.

Hydration Heroes:

- Water, herbal teas, and infused water are your best beverage buddies.

Foods to Avoid

Sugar Sabotage:

- Limit added sugars. Check labels for hidden sugar culprits.

- Minimize sugary beverages – your metabolism will thank you.

Processed Pitfalls:

- Say no to heavily processed foods with unpronounceable ingredients.

Sneaky Sodium:

- Keep an eye on sodium intake; excessive salt can disrupt metabolic balance.

Portion Control

Mindful Eating:

- Listen to your body's hunger and fullness cues.

- Use smaller plates to help manage portion sizes.

Protein Portioning:

- Distribute protein intake throughout the day for sustained muscle support.

Carb Conscious:

- Balance your carbohydrate intake based on activity levels.

Fats in Moderation:

- While healthy fats are essential, be mindful of portion sizes for overall calorie control.

CHAPTER 4

MEAL PLANNING AND RECIPES

Embarking on the Metabolic Reset Diet is not just a dietary shift; it's a lifestyle transformation that extends to every meal you consume. This chapter serves as your culinary guide, navigating through the intricacies of meal planning and offering a plethora of delectable recipes to ensure that your journey is not just health-conscious but also delightfully flavourful.

Sample Meal Plans for Different Phases

Diving into the Metabolic Reset Diet involves understanding the unique demands of each phase. Whether you're kickstarting your journey with the Initial Reset Phase or maintaining your newfound metabolic balance in the Maintenance Phase, here's a comprehensive breakdown to guide your meal planning.

Initial Reset Phase

The Initial Reset Phase is the launchpad for your metabolic transformation. During this phase, the focus is on cleansing your system and priming it for optimal functioning. Here's a sample meal plan to set you on the right track:

Day 1:

- **Breakfast:** Green Smoothie with Spinach, Kale, Banana, and Almond Milk

- **Snack:** Greek Yogurt with Berries

- **Lunch:** Grilled Chicken Salad with Mixed Greens and Olive Oil Dressing

- **Snack:** Sliced Cucumber with Hummus

- **Dinner:** Baked Salmon with Roasted Asparagus and Quinoa

Day 2:

- **Breakfast:** Oatmeal with Chia Seeds, Blueberries, and a Drizzle of Honey

- **Snack:** Apple Slices with Almond Butter

- **Lunch:** Turkey and Avocado Wrap with Whole Grain Tortilla

- **Snack:** Cherry Tomatoes with Mozzarella Cheese

- **Dinner:** Stir-Fried Tofu with Broccoli and Brown Rice

Day 3:

- **Breakfast:** Greek Yogurt Parfait with Mixed Berries and Granola

- **Snack:** Handful of Mixed Nuts (Almonds, Walnuts, Pistachios)
- **Lunch:** Quinoa Salad with Chickpeas, Tomatoes, Cucumbers, and Feta
- **Snack:** Carrot Sticks with Hummus
- **Dinner:** Grilled Shrimp with Quinoa and Steamed Asparagus

Day 4:

- **Breakfast:** Scrambled Eggs with Spinach and Tomatoes
- **Snack:** Cottage Cheese with Pineapple Chunks
- **Lunch:** Spinach and Feta Stuffed Chicken Breast with Roasted Sweet Potatoes
- **Snack:** Fresh Strawberries with Dark Chocolate Dipping Sauce
- **Dinner:** Baked Cod with Lemon Garlic Sauce, Quinoa, and Grilled Zucchini

Day 5:

- **Breakfast:** Smoothie Bowl with Acai, Mixed Berries, Banana, and Coconut Flakes

- **Snack:** Rice Cakes with Avocado Slices and Cherry Tomatoes

- **Lunch:** Lentil and Vegetable Soup with a Side of Whole Grain Bread

- **Snack:** Watermelon Cubes with Feta Cheese

- **Dinner:** Turkey Meatballs with Zucchini Noodles and Marinara Sauce

Day 6:

- **Breakfast:** Whole Grain Pancakes with Greek Yogurt and Fresh Mango

- **Snack:** Celery Sticks with Almond Butter

- **Lunch:** Grilled Vegetable and Quinoa Bowl with Balsamic Vinaigrette

- **Snack:** Orange Slices with Cottage Cheese

- **Dinner:** Baked Chicken Breast with Brussels Sprouts and Wild Rice

Day 7:

- **Breakfast:** Chia Seed Pudding with Coconut Milk and Mixed Berries

- **Snack:** Edamame Pods with Sea Salt

- **Lunch:** Mediterranean Chickpea Salad with Olives, Tomatoes, and Feta

- **Snack:** Pineapple and Mango Skewers

- **Dinner:** Stir-Fried Beef with Broccoli and Brown Rice

This phase is characterized by nutrient-dense, whole foods that support the detoxification process and kickstart your metabolism.

Maintenance Phase

As you transition to the Maintenance Phase, the emphasis shifts towards sustaining the positive changes achieved during the reset. Here's a sample meal plan designed to maintain metabolic balance:

Day 1:

- **Breakfast:** Quinoa Breakfast Bowl with Greek Yogurt, Nuts, and Fresh Fruit

- **Snack:** Celery Sticks with Peanut Butter

- **Lunch:** Shrimp and Vegetable Stir-Fry with Cauliflower Rice

- **Snack:** Mixed Berries Smoothie with Protein Powder

- **Dinner:** Grilled Steak with Sweet Potato Wedges and Steamed Broccoli

Day 2:

- **Breakfast:** Scrambled Eggs with Spinach and Feta Cheese

- **Snack:** Almonds and Dried Apricots

- **Lunch:** Chickpea Salad with Tomatoes, Cucumbers, and Feta

- **Snack:** Green Tea with a Slice of Lemon

- **Dinner:** Baked Cod with Lemon Garlic Sauce and Quinoa

Day 3:

- **Breakfast:** Overnight Oats with Chia Seeds, Almond Milk, and Fresh Berries

- **Snack:** Sliced Apple with Cheese

- **Lunch:** Turkey and Avocado Wrap with Whole Grain Tortilla

- **Snack:** Greek Yogurt Parfait with Granola

- **Dinner:** Stir-Fried Tofu with Broccoli and Brown Rice

Day 4:

- **Breakfast:** Whole Grain Pancakes with Maple Syrup and Sliced Bananas

- **Snack:** Carrot Sticks with Hummus

- **Lunch:** Quinoa and Black Bean Bowl with Avocado and Lime Dressing

- **Snack:** Mango and Pineapple Smoothie

- **Dinner:** Grilled Chicken Breast with Roasted Brussels Sprouts and Quinoa

Day 5:

- **Breakfast:** Smoked Salmon and Avocado Toast on Whole Grain Bread

- **Snack:** Mixed Nuts and Dark Chocolate

- **Lunch:** Mediterranean Salad with Feta, Olives, and Balsamic Vinaigrette

- **Snack:** Cottage Cheese with Pineapple

- **Dinner:** Baked Vegetable Lasagna with a Side Salad

Day 6:

- **Breakfast:** Blueberry and Spinach Smoothie Bowl with Almond Butter

- **Snack:** Rice Cakes with Cottage Cheese and Cherry Tomatoes

- **Lunch:** Lentil Soup with a Side of Whole Grain Bread

- **Snack:** Kiwi and Strawberry Fruit Salad

- **Dinner:** Pan-Seared Cod with Mango Salsa and Quinoa

Day 7:

- **Breakfast:** Egg White Omelette with Mushrooms, Spinach, and Feta

- **Snack:** Trail Mix with Dried Fruit

- **Lunch:** Grilled Vegetable Wrap with Hummus

- **Snack:** Pear Slices with Goat Cheese

- **Dinner:** Spaghetti Squash with Turkey Meatballs and Marinara Sauce

In the Maintenance Phase, the goal is to sustain a well-balanced diet that supports long-term health, incorporating a variety of nutrient-rich foods.

Recipe Ideas and Cooking Tips

Mastering the art of preparing delicious, metabolism-friendly meals is key to making the Metabolic Reset Diet a sustainable lifestyle. Here are some tantalizing recipe ideas and cooking tips for each major meal category:

Breakfast

Recipe 1: Avocado and Egg Breakfast Wrap

Ingredients:

- 1 whole-grain tortilla

- 1 ripe avocado, mashed

- 2 eggs, scrambled

- Salt and pepper to taste

- Fresh salsa for garnish

Instructions:

1. Heat the tortilla on a skillet until warm.

2. Spread the mashed avocado on the tortilla.

3. Scramble the eggs with salt and pepper and place them on the avocado.

4. Top with fresh salsa.

5. Fold the tortilla and enjoy a nutritious and filling breakfast.

Cooking Tips:

- Experiment with different salsas for varied flavors.

- Add a sprinkle of feta cheese for an extra burst of taste.

Recipe 2: Berry and Almond Overnight Oats

Ingredients:

- ½ cup rolled oats

- ½ cup almond milk

- ½ cup mixed berries (strawberries, blueberries, raspberries)

- 1 tablespoon almond butter

- 1 teaspoon honey

- Chopped nuts (almonds, walnuts) for topping

Instructions:

1. In a jar, combine rolled oats and almond milk.

2. Add mixed berries and stir well.

3. Seal the jar and refrigerate overnight.

4. In the morning, top with almond butter, a drizzle of honey, and chopped nuts.

5. Enjoy a delicious and nutrient-packed breakfast.

Cooking Tips:

- Customize by adding your favorite nuts or seeds.

- Experiment with different berries for variety.

Recipe 3: Spinach and Feta Egg Muffins

Ingredients:

- 6 eggs

- 1 cup fresh spinach, chopped

- ½ cup feta cheese, crumbled

- ¼ cup red bell pepper, diced

- Salt and pepper to taste

- Cooking spray for muffin tin

Instructions:

1. Preheat the oven to 350°F (175°C) and grease a muffin tin with cooking spray.

2. In a bowl, whisk eggs and season with salt and pepper.

3. Stir in chopped spinach, feta cheese, and diced red bell pepper.

4. Pour the mixture into the muffin tin, filling each cup.

5. Bake for 15-20 minutes until the egg muffins are set.

6. Allow them to cool slightly before removing from the tin.

7. Serve warm and savor a protein-rich breakfast.

Cooking Tips:

- Customize by adding other veggies like tomatoes or mushrooms.

- Make a batch ahead for quick and convenient breakfasts throughout the week.

Lunch

Recipe 1: Quinoa and Chickpea Salad Bowl

Ingredients:

- 1 cup cooked quinoa

- 1 cup canned chickpeas, drained and rinsed

- Cherry tomatoes, halved

- Cucumber, diced

- Red onion, finely chopped

- Feta cheese crumbles

- Olive oil and lemon dressing

Instructions:

1. In a bowl, combine quinoa, chickpeas, tomatoes, cucumber, and red onion.

2. Drizzle with olive oil and lemon dressing.

3. Toss well and top with feta cheese.

4. Enjoy a refreshing and protein-packed salad bowl.

Cooking Tips:

- Make a larger batch and store it for quick and convenient lunches throughout the week.

Recipe 2: Mediterranean Chicken and Hummus Wrap

Ingredients:

- Grilled chicken breast, thinly sliced

- Whole-grain wrap or tortilla

- Hummus

- Kalamata olives, sliced

- Red bell pepper, thinly sliced

- Baby spinach leaves

- Feta cheese, crumbled

- Extra virgin olive oil

Instructions:

1. Lay the whole-grain wrap on a clean surface.

2. Spread a generous layer of hummus across the center of the wrap.

3. Arrange the grilled chicken slices on top of the hummus.

4. Add Kalamata olives, sliced red bell pepper, and a handful of baby spinach leaves.

5. Sprinkle crumbled feta cheese over the ingredients.

6. Drizzle with extra virgin olive oil.

7. Fold the sides of the wrap and roll it tightly.

8. Slice in half and enjoy a Mediterranean-inspired, protein-packed wrap.

Cooking Tips:

- Experiment with flavored hummus for an extra burst of taste.

- Grill the chicken with Mediterranean spices like oregano and garlic for added flavor.

Recipe 3: Thai Quinoa Salad with Peanut Dressing

Ingredients:

- 1 cup cooked quinoa

- Shredded cooked chicken or tofu for a vegetarian option

- Shredded carrots

- Edamame beans, shelled

- Red cabbage, thinly sliced

- Fresh cilantro, chopped

- Peanuts, crushed

- Lime wedges

- Thai peanut dressing

Instructions:

1. In a large bowl, combine quinoa, shredded chicken or tofu, shredded carrots, edamame beans, and sliced red cabbage.

2. Drizzle with Thai peanut dressing and toss until well coated.

3. Top the salad with fresh cilantro and crushed peanuts.

4. Serve with lime wedges on the side for an extra zing.

5. Enjoy a vibrant and protein-rich Thai-inspired quinoa salad.

Cooking Tips:

- Prepare the Thai peanut dressing with a balance of sweet, salty, and tangy flavors.

- Customize the spice level by adjusting the amount of dressing used.

Additional Cooking Tips:

1. **Batch Preparation:** Consider preparing a larger quantity of the salads during your meal prep sessions. Divide them into individual containers for a hassle-free and nutritious lunch throughout the week.

2. **Ingredient Substitutions:** Don't hesitate to personalize the recipes based on your preferences or dietary restrictions. Substitute ingredients or add more veggies to suit your taste.

3. **Storage:** Store the prepared salads in airtight containers in the refrigerator. Keep any dressings or sauces separate until you're ready to enjoy the meal to maintain freshness.

Dinner

Recipe 1: Baked Salmon with Herb Crust

Ingredients:

- Salmon fillets

- Olive oil

- Fresh herbs (such as parsley, dill, and chives), finely chopped

- Lemon zest

- Salt and pepper

Instructions:

1. Preheat the oven to 375°F (190°C).

2. Place salmon fillets on a baking sheet.

3. Drizzle with olive oil and season with salt and pepper.

4. Mix chopped herbs and lemon zest, then press onto the salmon.

5. Bake for 15-20 minutes until the salmon is cooked through.

6. Serve with a side of roasted vegetables or quinoa.

Cooking Tips:

- Adjust herb quantities based on personal taste preferences.

- Squeeze fresh lemon juice over the salmon before serving for an extra burst of citrus flavour.

Recipe 2: Lemon Garlic Grilled Chicken with Quinoa

Ingredients:

- Chicken breasts

- Olive oil

- Garlic cloves, minced

- Lemon juice

- Fresh thyme leaves

- Salt and pepper

- Quinoa

Instructions:

1. **Marinate the Chicken:** In a bowl, combine olive oil, minced garlic, lemon juice, fresh thyme leaves, salt, and pepper. Marinate the chicken breasts in this flavorful mixture for at least 30 minutes.

2. **Preheat the Grill:** Ensure the grill is preheated to medium-high heat, providing the perfect environment for juicy and flavorful chicken.

3. **Grill the Chicken:** Place the marinated chicken breasts on the grill and cook for 6-8 minutes per side, or until the internal temperature reaches 165°F (74°C). The grill imparts a smoky flavor while maintaining the chicken's natural juiciness.

4. **Prepare Quinoa:** While the chicken is grilling, cook quinoa according to package instructions. Fluff it with a fork once done.

5. **Serve with Quinoa:** Plate the grilled chicken breasts alongside a serving of quinoa. Drizzle any remaining marinade over the chicken for an extra burst of flavor.

6. **Garnish and Enjoy:** Garnish with fresh thyme leaves and lemon wedges. The vibrant flavors of lemon and garlic will elevate the dish, making it a delightful and wholesome dinner option.

Recipe 3: Spiced Cauliflower Steaks with Turmeric Quinoa

Ingredients:

- Cauliflower heads, sliced into steaks

- Olive oil

- Ground cumin

- Ground coriander

- Smoked paprika

- Turmeric quinoa (cooked quinoa with added turmeric)

- Lemon wedges

- Fresh cilantro, chopped

- Salt and pepper

Instructions:

1. **Prepare Cauliflower Steaks:** Slice cauliflower heads into thick steaks. Brush each side with olive oil, ensuring an even coating.

2. **Create Spice Blend:** In a small bowl, mix ground cumin, ground coriander, smoked paprika, salt, and pepper to create a flavorful spice blend.

3. **Season Cauliflower:** Sprinkle the spice blend generously over the cauliflower steaks, ensuring they are well-coated with the aromatic spices.

4. **Roast the Cauliflower:** Place the seasoned cauliflower steaks on a baking sheet and roast in a preheated oven at 400°F (200°C) for 20-25 minutes or until the edges are golden and slightly crispy.

5. **Prepare Turmeric Quinoa:** While the cauliflower is roasting, cook quinoa with a dash of turmeric for vibrant colour and added anti-inflammatory benefits.

6. **Serve and Garnish:** Plate the spiced cauliflower steaks alongside a portion of turmeric quinoa. Drizzle with fresh lemon juice and garnish with chopped cilantro for a burst of freshness.

Snacks

Recipe 1: Greek Yogurt Parfait with Berries

Ingredients:

- Greek yogurt

- Mixed berries (strawberries, blueberries, raspberries)

- Granola

- Honey

Instructions:

1. In a glass or bowl, layer Greek yogurt at the bottom for a creamy base.

2. Add a generous layer of mixed berries for a burst of natural sweetness and antioxidants.

3. Sprinkle your favorite granola on top to introduce a satisfying crunch and additional fiber.

4. Drizzle the parfait with honey for a touch of sweetness and flavor enhancement.

5. Repeat the layers to create a visually appealing and delicious snack.

6. Dive in and savor the delightful combination of textures and flavors.

Cooking Tips:

- Opt for unsweetened Greek yogurt to control sugar intake while still enjoying the richness.

- Experiment with different types of granola, such as nut clusters or coconut flakes, to add varied textures and flavors.

Recipe 2: Nutty Banana Bites

Ingredients:

- Bananas, sliced

- Almond butter or peanut butter

- Chia seeds

- Walnuts or almonds, chopped

Instructions:

1. Spread a thin layer of almond or peanut butter on banana slices.

2. Sprinkle chia seeds on top for an extra nutrient boost and a subtle crunch.

3. Garnish with chopped walnuts or almonds for a satisfying blend of textures and flavors.

4. Arrange the banana bites on a plate or tray.

5. Refrigerate for a few minutes to allow the nut butter to slightly firm up.

6. Indulge in these nutrient-packed banana bites for a quick and energizing snack.

Cooking Tips:

- Choose ripe but firm bananas for the best texture and sweetness.

- Customize with a drizzle of honey or a sprinkle of cinnamon for added sweetness and warmth.

Recipe 3: Veggie and Hummus Platter

Ingredients:

- Baby carrots

- Cherry tomatoes

- Cucumber, sliced

- Bell pepper strips (assorted colors)

- Hummus

Instructions:

1. Arrange baby carrots, cherry tomatoes, cucumber slices, and bell pepper strips on a platter.

2. Place a bowl of hummus in the center for dipping.

3. Dive into this colorful and crunchy snack, pairing the freshness of veggies with the creamy goodness of hummus.

Cooking Tips:

- Experiment with homemade hummus flavors, such as roasted red pepper or garlic and herb.

- Pre-cut and store the veggies in portioned containers for a convenient grab-and-go option.

CHAPTER 5

EXERCISE AND PHYSICAL ACTIVITY

In this chapter, we dive deep into the pivotal role of exercise and physical activity within the Metabolic Reset Diet. As you've embarked on this transformative journey, it's crucial to recognize that a holistic approach to health involves not just dietary modifications but an integration of movement that synergizes with your metabolic reset goals.

Integration of Exercise with the Metabolic Reset Diet

In the Metabolic Reset Diet, exercise isn't just an afterthought; it's a fundamental pillar that complements and amplifies the benefits of dietary changes. The integration of exercise into your routine serves as a catalyst for metabolic recalibration, supporting weight loss, enhancing insulin sensitivity, and promoting overall well-being.

Understanding the Symbiosis: Diet and Exercise Harmony

Think of your body as a high-performance machine, and the Metabolic Reset Diet as the premium fuel it needs. Now, imagine exercise as the engine that optimizes the utilization of this fuel, propelling you towards your health and fitness goals. The synergy between diet and exercise is not just advantageous; it's transformative.

By engaging in regular physical activity, you create an environment where the body becomes more receptive to the metabolic changes induced by the diet. Exercise amplifies the metabolic effects, fostering an efficient and resilient system that can adapt to the new nutritional paradigm. This symbiosis ensures that your metabolic reset isn't just effective; it's sustainable.

Recommended Types of Exercise

Now that we've established the importance of exercise let's delve into the specifics. The Metabolic Reset Diet encourages a well-rounded approach to physical activity, encompassing various forms of exercise to address different facets of your health.

Aerobic Exercise: Elevating Heart Health and Fat Burning

Aerobic exercise, often referred to as cardio, is a cornerstone in the Metabolic Reset journey. It's not just about sweating it out; it's about elevating your heart rate and improving cardiovascular health. Whether it's brisk walking, running, cycling, or dancing, aerobic exercises stimulate the cardiovascular system, enhancing blood flow and oxygen delivery to tissues.

In the context of metabolic resetting, aerobic exercise plays a dual role. First, it promotes fat burning, aiding in weight loss and the mobilization of stored energy. Second, it enhances insulin sensitivity, a key factor in metabolic health. Regular aerobic sessions improve the body's ability to regulate blood sugar, a crucial aspect of the metabolic reset process.

Strength Training: Sculpting Your Metabolic Machinery

Strength training is the sculptor of your metabolic landscape. Far from just building muscle for aesthetics, it plays a pivotal role in the Metabolic Reset Diet by boosting your metabolism and supporting sustainable weight loss.

When you engage in strength training, whether through weight lifting, resistance exercises, or bodyweight workouts, you're not just building muscle mass. You're creating a metabolic furnace that continues to burn calories even at rest. More muscle equates to a higher basal metabolic rate (BMR), contributing to the overall effectiveness of your metabolic reset.

Importance of Regular Physical Activity

Exercise isn't just a means to an end; it's a lifestyle. Regular physical activity goes beyond the confines of a gym session; it permeates your daily routine, becoming an integral part of your life. The Metabolic Reset Diet acknowledges the importance of this consistent movement for sustained well-being.

Balancing Hormones and Mood Enhancement

Regular physical activity is a natural regulator of hormones, including those responsible for stress and mood. As you traverse the ups and downs of life, exercise becomes your ally in maintaining hormonal balance, reducing stress, and uplifting your mood. This emotional resilience is a crucial component of a successful metabolic reset journey.

Enhanced Sleep Quality

Exercise isn't just about what happens during the workout; it extends its benefits into the realm of sleep. Quality sleep is a cornerstone of metabolic health, and regular physical activity contributes to improved sleep patterns. As you engage in the Metabolic Reset Diet, the synergy between exercise and sleep becomes a powerful ally in optimizing your body's metabolic processes.

Optimizing Metabolism for the Long Haul

The Metabolic Reset Diet isn't a sprint; it's a marathon towards lasting health. Regular physical activity ensures that your metabolism remains dynamic and responsive. It guards against stagnation, preventing plateaus and ensuring that your metabolic machinery operates at its peak efficiency.

Crafting Your Exercise Routine: Personalization is Key

As you integrate exercise into your Metabolic Reset journey, remember that personalization is the key to sustainability. Tailor your workouts to your preferences, fitness levels, and any existing health considerations. The goal is to create a routine that not only aligns with the metabolic reset principles but also brings you joy and fulfillment.

CHAPTER 6

MONITORING AND ADJUSTMENTS

In this chapter, we embark on a comprehensive exploration of the nuanced art of monitoring progress and making thoughtful adjustments. The success of your journey hinges on your ability to navigate the seas of change, adapting your course based on the ever-shifting currents of your body's response to the Metabolic Reset Diet.

Tracking Progress: Unveiling the Map of Your Transformation

Embarking on the Metabolic Reset Diet is akin to setting sail on a voyage of self-discovery and renewal. To steer your ship effectively, you need a reliable map – a system that goes beyond mere weight management, providing insights into the multifaceted changes unfolding within.

Weight Management: Beyond the Numbers

The scale, while a tangible metric, often fails to capture the intricate nuances of your metabolic journey. Weight management in the Metabolic Reset Diet extends beyond numerical values on a scale. It's about deciphering changes in body composition, understanding shifts in energy levels, and appreciating the overall enhancement of well-being. Incorporate diverse metrics such as body fat percentage, measurements, and the fit of your clothes to construct a comprehensive narrative of your transformative odyssey.

Other Health Indicators: The Holistic View

The Metabolic Reset Diet is a holistic endeavor, aiming to optimize not just weight but overall health. Beyond the scale, monitor key health indicators that offer a panoramic view of your well-being. Keep a watchful eye on blood pressure, cholesterol levels, and markers of inflammation. These indicators serve as compass points, guiding you toward a deeper understanding of how your body responds to the metabolic reset.

Making Adjustments to the Diet: Navigating the Waters of Adaptation

As your metabolic ship sails through the waves of change, it's essential to navigate the inevitable currents and winds of adjustment. Skilfully adapting your dietary strategy ensures that you not only stay on course but flourish amidst the evolving needs of your unique physiology.

Plateau Management: Breaking Through Barriers

Plateaus, akin to islands in your journey, are a common feature in any transformative process, including the Metabolic Reset Diet. A plateau doesn't signal an impending storm but rather a call to recalibrate your course. Explore strategies such as adjusting calorie intake, diversifying your exercise routine, or embracing intermittent fasting to reignite the flames of your metabolism. Plateaus are not roadblocks but invitations to explore uncharted territories.

Adapting to Individual Needs: The Personalized Approach

The Metabolic Reset Diet is not a rigid set of rules; it's a flexible framework designed to adapt to the uniqueness of each individual. Embrace the power of personalization. If certain foods or strategies don't resonate with your body, consider it an opportunity for fine-tuning. Experiment with different food combinations, explore alternative exercise routines, and attune yourself to your body's cues. In the realm of metabolic resetting, individualization is the compass that guides you towards lasting success.

Crafting Your Monitoring and Adjustment Strategy: The Captain's Log

As you set sail into the realm of monitoring and adjustment, envision yourself as the captain of your metabolic ship. Craft a personalized strategy that aligns with your goals and resonates with your preferences. Consider maintaining a journal, your Captain's Log, to document daily experiences, challenges, and victories. Regularly reassess your goals, celebrate milestones, and proactively make adjustments based on your evolving understanding of your body's signals.

Chapter 7

POTENTIAL BENEFITS AND RISKS

Welcome to Chapter 7, where we embark on a thorough exploration of the Metabolic Reset Diet's potential benefits and considerate reflections on associated risks. As you navigate through the seas of metabolic transformation, it's essential to understand the terrain, appreciating the rewards that await while being mindful of the challenges that may arise.

Positive Outcomes of the Metabolic Reset Diet

The Metabolic Reset Diet isn't just a regimen; it's a transformative odyssey that holds the potential for a myriad of positive outcomes. Let's illuminate the landscape of benefits that await those who embark on this journey.

Enhanced Weight Management: Beyond the Numbers

At the forefront of positive outcomes lies enhanced weight management. The Metabolic Reset Diet, when diligently followed, offers a pathway to shedding excess pounds. However, its essence extends beyond numerical values on a scale. It's about fostering a sustainable relationship with food, addressing the root causes of weight fluctuations, and embracing a healthier body composition.

Improved Insulin Sensitivity: A Key to Metabolic Health

A significant triumph of the Metabolic Reset Diet is the improvement of insulin sensitivity. By harmonizing dietary choices with metabolic needs, this approach supports the body in regulating blood sugar levels effectively. Enhanced insulin sensitivity not only aids in weight management but also contributes to the prevention of metabolic disorders, laying the foundation for enduring health.

Reduction in Inflammation: Soothing the Body's Symphony

Inflammation, often a silent culprit in various health issues, is addressed by the Metabolic Reset Diet. By prioritizing nutrient-dense foods and minimizing inflammatory triggers, this dietary approach seeks to create a harmonious internal environment. The result? A reduction in inflammation, promoting overall well-being and mitigating the risk of chronic diseases.

Potential Risks and Considerations

While the Metabolic Reset Diet holds promises of transformative benefits, it's prudent to navigate the seas with awareness of potential risks and considerations. Let's delve into these waters with a discerning eye.

Health Precautions: Navigating Individual Health Profiles

Individual health profiles vary, and certain conditions may warrant caution when undertaking the Metabolic Reset Diet. It's crucial to consider factors such as pre-existing medical conditions, medications, and individual health history. Consulting with a healthcare professional before embarking on this journey ensures that your metabolic reset aligns with your unique health needs.

Common Challenges and How to Overcome Them: Steadying the Course

Every voyage encounters storms, and the Metabolic Reset journey is no exception. Common challenges, such as dietary adjustments, cravings, and navigating social situations, may arise. Acknowledging these challenges and proactively seeking solutions ensures a smoother voyage. Incorporating mindfulness practices, enlisting support from friends or online communities, and staying flexible in your approach are strategies to navigate these common challenges.

Crafting Your Approach: A Balanced Perspective

As you navigate the potential benefits and considerations in Chapter 7, it's essential to adopt a balanced perspective. Embrace the positive outcomes with enthusiasm, recognizing the transformative potential of the Metabolic Reset Diet. Simultaneously, approach potential risks with awareness, taking proactive steps to mitigate challenges and ensuring that your journey is not just transformative but also sustainable.

Chapter 8

SCIENTIFIC RESEARCH AND STUDIES

Welcome to Chapter 8, a journey into the heart of the Metabolic Reset Diet. In this chapter, we explore the bedrock upon which this transformative approach stands – scientific research and studies. The fusion of ancient wisdom and contemporary science not only validates the efficacy of the Metabolic Reset Diet but also propels it into the realm of evidence-based health.

Recent Studies on Metabolic Reset

To comprehend the significance of the Metabolic Reset Diet, we delve into the latest scientific research that illuminates its principles and outcomes. These studies serve as beacons, guiding us through the empirical landscape of metabolic resetting.

Unravelling the Metabolic Mechanisms

Recent studies dissect the intricate mechanisms through which the Metabolic Reset Diet influences the body. From hormonal modulation to gene expression, scientific inquiry reveals the physiological transformations that underpin the diet's effectiveness. Understanding these mechanisms not only fortifies the diet's credibility but also equips practitioners with profound insights into their own metabolic processes.

Metabolic Reset and Chronic Conditions

Scientific exploration extends beyond weight management, investigating the impact of the Metabolic Reset Diet on chronic conditions. Studies explore its role in mitigating factors associated with metabolic syndrome, type 2 diabetes, and cardiovascular health. The findings herald a paradigm shift, positioning the diet not only as a weight loss strategy but as a holistic approach to addressing underlying health concerns.

Scientific Support and Criticisms

As we navigate the scientific seas, it's essential to acknowledge the presence of both advocates and skeptics. This section scrutinizes the scientific landscape, weighing the support and criticisms that surround the Metabolic Reset Diet.

Advocacy: Voices in Support

In the realm of scientific support, voices resonate with the positive outcomes of the Metabolic Reset Diet. Advocates highlight the alignment of its principles with fundamental physiological processes. They underscore the adaptability of the diet, emphasizing its potential to cater to diverse individual needs. Scientific endorsements act as pillars, reinforcing the credibility of the Metabolic Reset approach.

Criticisms: Navigating Controversies

No scientific inquiry is immune to criticism, and the Metabolic Reset Diet is no exception. This section addresses controversies and critiques, examining concerns raised by skeptics. Whether questioning the long-term sustainability of the diet or probing into potential side effects, a balanced exploration of criticisms fosters a comprehensive understanding of the Metabolic Reset landscape.

Crafting Your Informed Perspective: A Symbiosis of Wisdom

As you delve into the scientific realms of Chapter 8, bear in mind that knowledge is your compass. In navigating the Metabolic Reset Diet, draw upon both ancient wisdom and contemporary science. Acknowledge the robust support while remaining vigilant to criticisms, and let this symbiosis guide your informed perspective.

SUCCESS STORIES AND TESTIMONIALS

Welcome to the heart of Chapter 9, where the tapestry of the Metabolic Reset Diet comes alive through the vivid narratives of individuals who have embarked on this transformative journey. These success stories and testimonials illuminate the path ahead, showcasing the tangible impact of the Metabolic Reset Diet on real lives.

Real-life Experiences with the Metabolic Reset Diet: Stories of Transformation

In this section, we invite you to delve into the intimate and authentic narratives of individuals who have embraced the Metabolic Reset Diet and emerged on the other side with remarkable stories of transformation.

1. Tom's Journey: From Fatigue to Fulfillment

Meet Tom, a 42-year-old professional juggling the demands of a high-stakes career and family life. Before discovering the Metabolic Reset Diet, Tom found himself trapped in a cycle of fatigue and stress. His sedentary lifestyle and reliance on quick, processed meals took a toll on his energy levels and overall well-being.

Tom's introduction to the Metabolic Reset Diet was a turning point. As he gradually adopted the diet's principles, incorporating nutrient-dense foods and engaging in regular physical activity, a remarkable shift occurred. Tom not only shed excess weight but experienced a surge in energy levels that transformed his professional and personal life. His story underscores the profound impact of the Metabolic Reset Diet on holistic well-being.

2. Emily's Triumph: Conquering Emotional Eating

Emily's journey with the Metabolic Reset Diet is a testament to the transformative power of mindful eating. Struggling with emotional eating and its impact on her weight, Emily found solace and guidance in the principles of the Metabolic Reset Diet.

Through the diet's emphasis on nourishing the body and fostering a healthy relationship with food, Emily learned to listen to her body's cues and break free from the chains of emotional eating. Her journey not only resulted in weight loss but, more importantly, restored her sense of control and self-empowerment.

Transformative Journeys and Lessons Learned: Beyond the Scale

In this segment, we explore the broader lessons gleaned from these transformative journeys, transcending the numerical values on the scale.

Lesson 1: Mindful Eating as a Lifestyle

The stories of individuals like Emily highlight the pivotal role of mindful eating in the Metabolic Reset Diet. It's not just about the food on your plate; it's about the relationship you forge with every bite. By cultivating mindfulness, individuals discover a profound connection with their bodies and a newfound ability to make choices that align with their well-being.

Lesson 2: Sustainability and Adaptability

Both Tom and Emily's experiences underscore the sustainability and adaptability inherent in the Metabolic Reset Diet. It's not a rigid set of rules but a dynamic framework that adjusts to individual needs. Sustainability is not just about reaching a goal; it's about creating a lifestyle that supports lasting health and vitality.

Lesson 3: Community and Support

Across these narratives, a common thread emerges – the importance of community and support. Whether it's a partner, friends, or an online community, the Metabolic Reset Diet thrives when individuals share their experiences and support one another. This sense of shared journey becomes a source of inspiration, motivation, and resilience.

Expert Insights and Practical Takeaways: Bridging Stories with Science

In this section, we bridge the real-life narratives with expert insights, providing practical takeaways for readers.

Insight 1: Individualization is Key

The stories of Tom and Emily emphasize that one size does not fit all. The Metabolic Reset Diet's effectiveness lies in its ability to be tailored to individual needs. Understanding and adapting to your unique physiology ensures a more personalized and successful journey.

Insight 2: The Emotional Aspect of Eating Matters

Emily's journey sheds light on the emotional aspect of eating. The Metabolic Reset Diet recognizes that addressing emotional eating is crucial for long-term success. Building a positive relationship with food is not just about what you eat but also why and how you eat.

Insight 3: Celebrate Non-Scale Victories

While weight loss is a common goal, Tom and Emily's stories remind us to celebrate non-scale victories. Increased energy, improved mood, and enhanced overall well-being are equally significant markers of success on the Metabolic Reset journey.

Inspiring Tomorrow's Success Stories

As we conclude this chapter, the real-life stories shared here are more than testimonials; they are beacons of hope and inspiration. The Metabolic Reset Diet is not just a roadmap; it's a vessel that carries individuals towards a brighter, healthier future. May these stories serve as guiding lights, illuminating the path for those who embark on their own transformative journey with the Metabolic Reset Diet.

Chapter 10

CHARTING A COURSE TO LASTING WELLNESS WITH THE METABOLIC RESET DIET

As we navigate the expansive seas of health and well-being, the Metabolic Reset Diet emerges not just as a dietary strategy but as a transformative journey towards lasting vitality. In this conclusion, we'll embark on a reflective voyage, exploring the key takeaways, envisioning future trends, and celebrating the profound shift in perspective that the Metabolic Reset Diet invites.

Unveiling the Tapestry of Health

The Metabolic Reset Diet, as we've explored in preceding chapters, is not a mere set of rules but a dynamic approach that intertwines with the intricacies of individual metabolism. It's a tapestry woven with the threads of personalized nutrition, mindful movement, and a commitment to overall well-being.

Acknowledging the Transformative Power

At its core, the Metabolic Reset Diet is more than a means to shed pounds; it's a catalyst for a comprehensive metamorphosis. The stories of individuals who have embraced this journey serve as living testimonies to its transformative power. From reclaiming vitality and hormonal balance to navigating challenges with resilience, these narratives illustrate that the Metabolic Reset Diet transcends the realm of traditional diets, becoming a lifestyle that permeates every facet of life.

Holistic Approach to Wellness

What sets the Metabolic Reset Diet apart is its holistic approach to wellness. It doesn't isolate weight loss as the sole marker of success; rather, it emphasizes optimizing overall health. The integration of exercise, the focus on mindful eating, and the acknowledgment of emotional and mental well-being underscore a paradigm shift – health is not just a physical state; it's a holistic equilibrium.

Key Takeaways: Lessons from the Metabolic Reset Journey

As we stand at the conclusion of this exploration, let's distill the key takeaways that illuminate the path to success with the Metabolic Reset Diet.

1. Personalization is the Key

The Metabolic Reset Diet is not a one-size-fits-all solution. It thrives on personalization, recognizing that each individual's metabolism is as unique as their fingerprint.

From tailoring dietary choices to adapting exercise routines, the power lies in the ability to fine-tune the approach based on individual needs and responses.

2. Mindful Eating Nourishes Body and Soul

Beyond the nutritional content of food, the Metabolic Reset Diet invites a deeper connection with eating through mindfulness. Conscious choices, savoring each bite, and being attuned to hunger and fullness – these practices not only support weight management but foster a harmonious relationship with food.

3. Exercise is a Joyful Journey

In the realm of the Metabolic Reset Diet, exercise is not a punitive measure but a joyful journey. Whether it's aerobic activities, strength training, or simply incorporating movement into daily life, the emphasis is on finding activities that bring pleasure. Exercise becomes a celebration of what the body can achieve, a source of energy and vitality.

4. Adaptability is the Cornerstone of Progress

The journey with the Metabolic Reset Diet is not a linear path; it's a dynamic expedition with twists and turns. Those who navigate setbacks with adaptability, recalibrating their course when needed, find sustained progress. The ability to adjust dietary strategies, tweak exercise routines, and respond to the evolving needs of the body is a hallmark of success.

5. Holistic Health is the True Victory

Weight loss, while a visible marker, is just one facet of success with the Metabolic Reset Diet. The true victory lies in achieving holistic health – optimized metabolism, hormonal balance, mental clarity, and emotional well-being. Success stories reveal that individuals often discover benefits beyond their initial expectations, redefining their understanding of what it means to be truly healthy.

Future Trends and Developments in Metabolic Reset Diets

As we bid farewell to the Metabolic Reset Diet of 2024, let's cast our gaze towards the horizon, envisioning future trends and developments in the realm of metabolic health.

Advances in Personalized Nutrition

The future of metabolic reset diets is poised to witness a surge in personalized nutrition. With advancements in genetic testing, data analytics, and a deeper understanding of individual responses to different foods, metabolic reset strategies will likely become increasingly tailored to the unique genetic and metabolic makeup of each individual.

Integration of Technology for Monitoring and Guidance

Technology, with its ever-evolving capabilities, will play a central role in the future of metabolic reset diets. From wearable devices that track metabolic markers to sophisticated apps providing real-time guidance, individuals will have unprecedented tools at their disposal for monitoring progress and receiving personalized recommendations.

Holistic Wellness as a Cultural Shift

The Metabolic Reset Diet is not just a trend; it's indicative of a broader cultural shift towards embracing holistic wellness. As individuals recognize the interconnectedness of physical, mental, and emotional well-being, the demand for lifestyle approaches that address the entirety of health will continue to grow.

CONCLUSION

YOUR JOURNEY, YOUR LEGACY

In conclusion, the Metabolic Reset Diet is not just a chapter in the book of health and well-being; it's a narrative that you, as an individual, are writing. Your journey is a testament to the potential for transformation that resides within each choice you make – from the foods you nourish your body with to the movements that invigorate your spirit.

As you traverse the seas of health, remember that the Metabolic Reset Diet is not a destination; it's a journey, an exploration of your body's potential for enduring vitality. Embrace the lessons learned, celebrate the victories, and carry forward the principles of personalization, mindfulness, adaptability, and holistic well-being into every chapter of your life.

Your journey with the Metabolic Reset Diet is not just for you; it's a legacy that ripples through the lives of those around you, inspiring others to embark on their own quests for health and vitality. As the captain of your ship, chart your course with intention, navigate challenges with resilience, and let the winds of well-being carry you towards a legacy of lasting health and vitality. Bon voyage!